Vegetarian Cookbook

Healthy, Easy and Delicious
Vegetarian Recipes for Weight Loss

Angelica Auton

Table of Contents

CHAPTER 3

DINNER RECIPES 53

CHAPTER 4

SIDE RECIPES 77

CHAPTER 5

DESSERT RECIPES 98

Introduction

A vegetarian Diet is a lifestyle based on enjoying plant-based food and having meals without meat, fish or poultry. Followers are often called "vegans" because they not only avoid meat products but also avoid other animal products such as dairy and eggs, and leather and wool in clothing.

Being vegetarian is not just a diet choice but also a way of life. Most people think that a vegetarian lifestyle means limiting or avoiding all kinds of food, but it does not have to be so. Vegetarians can include dairy products, eggs and some types of fish in their diet, as long as they don't contain meat sources. Here I provide an overview of the vegetarian diet so you know what you are getting into when you decide to become vegetarian.

Where did Vegetarianism Originate?

Vegetarianism is based on religious dietary rules established by the Jewish religion more than 3,500 years ago for Passover and biblical festivals. Tradition says that God created the world with plants and animals, but God didn't want them to eat each other. So, the prophet Moses told Aaron to get wood that could burn completely without leaving any soot, and Aaron crafted an altar where people could not bring any meat or fish. When Moses died, his followers missed meat, so they brought lamb and offered it on the altars. When they realized that God doesn't like the idea of worshipping with meat, they stopped offering the lamb. From that story came the vegetarian tradition.

The term "vegetarian" was originally used in the 18th century to describe a diet without meat, and it was promoted by a movement created by the Indian leader, Mohandas Gandhi. He tried to convince people that animal slaughtering was wrong for many reasons: religious, economic, social and ecologic.

Historically, vegetarianism has been promoted as a healthy diet because it reduces the chances for many diseases such as cardiovascular disease and cancer. In addition, vegetarians live longer than non-vegetarians and suffer less from chronic illnesses such as diabetes and heart disease.

Becoming a Vegetarian

There are many reasons why people choose vegetarianism as a lifestyle.

- Religious – most religions promote vegetarian diets as part of their teachings.
- Environmental – a vegetarian diet is more sustainable as a result of less use of the world's resources, and it reduces the greenhouse gases that lead to global warming.
- Economical – vegetarians don't have to spend money on meat products, which can be expensive. In addition, eating high-quality fresh produce is much cheaper than consuming meat products.

Where do you start? If you're considering becoming vegetarian, I suggest you start gradually and establish your goals clearly so you don't give up easily.

Should to go Vegetarian?

Many people think that today, vegetarian diets are the healthiest for humans. In addition, global health care standards suggest a balanced diet that contains all the necessary nutrients and includes all food categories. Unfortunately, a vegetarian diet is not the ideal diet for every person. It may not be enough to fulfill your daily nutritional needs because it lacks several important sources of nutrition: iron, calcium, zinc and B12.

A vegetarian diet also changes your will power (and often a lot of it), but the results are worth the effort. The benefits are worth it!

All the best on the healthy path you have chosen to follow.

Breakfast

Recipes

1. Carrot Quinoa Power Muffins

Preparation Time: 20 minutes

Cooking Time: 18 minutes

Servings: 18

Ingredients:

1 cup cooked quinoa, cooled

1 cup grated carrot

2 large eggs, beaten

¾ cup coconut sugar

½ cup chopped pecans

½ cup melted coconut oil

½ cup plain nonfat Greek yogurt

1 teaspoon vanilla extract

¾ cup plus 1 tablespoon wholewheat flour

¾ cup plus 1 tablespoon almond flour

1 tablespoon chia seeds

1 tablespoon sesame seeds

1 teaspoon baking soda

½ teaspoon salt

Directions:

- Preheat the oven to 350°F. Line two muffin tins with 18 liners and set aside.
- In a large bowl, stir together the quinoa, carrot, eggs, coconut sugar, pecans, coconut oil, yogurt, and vanilla.
- In a medium bowl, stir together the wholewheat flour, almond flour, chia seeds, sesame seeds, baking soda, and salt.
- Stir the flour mixture into the quinoa mixture to combine. Evenly divide the batter among the prepared liners, filling each three-fourths full.
- Bake for 18 minutes, until lightly browned on top. Remove and let cool.
- Put 2 muffins into each of 9 single-serving 24-ounce meal prep containers or quart-size resealable bags. Refrigerate for up to 5 days.

Nutrition:

Calories: 185

Fat: 12g

Protein: 3g

Total carbs: 18g

Net carbs: 16g

Fiber: 2g

Sugar: 10g

Sodium: 162mg

2. Pumpkin Chocolate Chip Waffles

Preparation Time: 10 minutes

Cooking Time: 5 minutes

Servings: 6

Ingredients:

2 cups wholewheat flour

2 teaspoons ground cinnamon

2 teaspoons baking powder

¼ teaspoon salt

1 (15-ounce) can pumpkin purée

1 cup unsweetened almond milk

¼ cup olive oil

1 tablespoon raw honey

½ cup mini semisweet chocolate chips

Nonstick cooking spray

Directions:

- Preheat a waffle iron according to the manufacturer's instructions.

- In a medium bowl, stir together the flour, cinnamon, baking powder, and salt.
- In another medium bowl, whisk the pumpkin, almond milk, olive oil, and honey until blended.
- Slowly pour the pumpkin mixture into the flour mixture and stir until well incorporated. Stir in the chocolate chips.
- Coat the waffle iron with cooking spray.
- Add ¾ cup of batter to the iron. Cook each waffle for 3 to 4 minutes. Set aside to cool.
- Repeat with the remaining batter.
- Put 1 waffle into each of 6 quart-size resealable bags.
- Refrigerate for up to 5 days.

Nutrition:

Calories: 366

Fat: 17g

Protein: 8g

Total carbs: 54g

Net carbs: 45g

Fiber: 9g

Sugar: 16g

Sodium: 162mg

3. **Vegetable Egg Muffins**

Preparation Time: 10 minutes

Cooking Time: 30 minutes

Servings: 18 muffins

Ingredients:

Nonstick cooking spray

6 large eggs

1 (16-ounce) carton egg whites

1½ cups shredded russet potato

1¼ cups meatless crumbles (such as Boca brand)

1 cup chopped bell pepper, any color

½ cup shredded pepper Jack cheese

¼ teaspoon salt

¼ teaspoon freshly ground black pepper

Directions:

- Preheat the oven to 350°F. Coat two muffin tins with cooking spray and set aside.
- In a large bowl, whisk the whole eggs and egg whites for 30 seconds, until fluffy. Pour ¼ cup of the egg mixture into each of 18 muffin tin wells.

- In a medium bowl, stir together the potato, crumbles, bell pepper, Jack cheese, salt, and pepper. Distribute the potato filling evenly on top of the egg filling.
- Bake for 30 minutes, or until the centers are firm and a toothpick inserted into the center of a muffin comes out clean. Remove and let cool.
- Put 3 muffins into each of 6 quart-size resealable bags. Refrigerate for up to 5 days.

Nutrition:

Calories: 181

Fat: 8g

Protein: 20g

Total carbs: 7g

Net carbs: 6g

Fiber: 1g

Sugar: 2g

Sodium: 359mg

4. Zucchini Bagel Sandwich

Preparation Time: 25 minutes

Cooking Time: 17 minutes

Servings: 4

Ingredients:

Nonstick cooking spray

3 cups grated zucchini

1 cup shredded mozzarella cheese

1/3 cup coconut flour

1 teaspoon baking powder

¼ teaspoon sea salt

2 large eggs

1 cup egg whites

1 tablespoon hot sauce

Directions:

- Preheat the oven to 400°F. Spray a donut mold with cooking spray.
- Put the grated zucchini in a colander in the sink and let drain for 20 minutes.
- Transfer to a cheesecloth or multiple paper towels and squeeze out all the excess moisture. The zucchini should be very dry.

- In a small microwaveable bowl, heat the mozzarella cheese in 30-second increments until melted.
- In a large bowl, stir together the coconut flour, drained zucchini, baking powder, salt, and whole eggs.
- Add the melted mozzarella and mix with your clean hands until a dough form. Evenly divide the dough among 4 cavities of the mold.
- Bake for 15 to 17 minutes, until the bagels are completely set with no sign of jiggling. Remove and let cool.
- Turn the pan upside-down and shake to remove the bagels onto a plate. Set aside.
- Heat a medium nonstick skillet over medium heat. Add the egg whites and cook for 3 to 4 minutes, without stirring, or until no longer shiny and runny.
- Fold the eggs in half and flip. Cook for 1 minute more. Remove the eggs from the skillet and cut into 4 squares. Drizzle each piece lightly with hot sauce. Set aside to cool.
- Place 1 bagel and 1 egg white square into each of 4 single-serving 24-ounce meal prep containers or quart-size resealable bags. Refrigerate for up to 5 days.

Nutrition:

Calories: 253

Fat: 10g

Protein: 21g

Total carbs: 20g

Net carbs: 10g

Fiber: 10g

Sugar: 2g

Sodium: 418mg

5. **Sweet Potato Pancakes**

Preparation Time: 10 minutes

Cooking Time: 10 minutes

Servings: 2

Ingredients:

1 cup cooked, mashed peeled sweet potato

1 cup egg whites

1 teaspoon ground cinnamon

½ teaspoon ground ginger

½ teaspoon ground allspice

½ teaspoon salt

Nonstick cooking spray

3 tablespoons smooth almond butter

3 tablespoons sugar-free pancake syrup or pure maple syrup

Directions:

- Heat a griddle or large skillet over medium heat.
- In a large bowl, stir together the mashed sweet potato and egg whites until blended.
- Stir in the cinnamon, ginger, allspice, and salt.
- Spray the griddle with cooking spray.

- Using a 1/3-cup measure, scoop the batter onto the griddle. This should make 6 pancakes (you may have to work in batches).
- Cook for 2 to 3 minutes, flip the pancakes, and cook for about 1 minute more, until slightly browned. Remove from the skillet and let cool on a plate.
- In each of the 2 (2-ounce) containers, put 1½ tablespoons of almond butter. In each of the 2 separate (2-ounce) containers, put 1½ tablespoons of syrup.
- Put 3 pancakes into each of 2 single-serving 24-ounce meal prep containers.
- Add 1 almond butter container and 1 syrup container to each pancake container. Refrigerate for up to 5 days.

Nutrition:

Calories: 384

Fat: 14g

Protein: 21g

Total carbs: 48g

Net carbs: 41g

Fiber: 7g

Sugar: 26g

Sodium: 644mg

6. Whole Food Smoothie

Preparation Time: 10 minutes

Cooking Time: 0 minutes

Servings: 4

Ingredients:

Kiwi – 1, leave peel on

Baby zucchini – ½, leave peel on

Pineapple – ¼, peel removed

Green or white grapes – 1 cup

Kale leaves – 4, stemmed

Fresh strawberries – 4, including green tops

Lime – 1 thin slice, leave peel on

Peeled orange – ½

Banana – ½ peeled

Small handful wheatgrass

Spirulina – 1 Tbsp.

Kelp granules – 1 Tbsp.

Flaxseed – 1 Tbsp.

Coldwater – 1 cup

Ice – 1 cup

Directions:

- Add all the ingredients in a blender, starting with fruits and vegetables then spirulina, kelp, and flaxseed.
- Lastly, add the water and ice.
- Blend for 1 minute and serve.

Nutrition:

Calories: 132

Fat: 1g

Carb: 25g

Protein: 3g

7. Amaranth Oat Waffles

Preparation Time: 15 minutes

Cooking Time: 25 minutes

Servings: 8

Ingredients:

Dry ingredients

Whole grain amaranth flour – 1 cup

Oat flour – ½ cup

Oat bran – ½ cup

Whole soy flour – ½ cup

Whole grain corn flour – ½ cup

Whole grain coarse cornmeal – ¼ cup

Flax meal – 2 Tbsp.

Baking powder – 2 ½ tsp.

Baking soda – ½ tsp.

Pinch sea salt

Wet ingredients

Equal parts of soy or almond milk – 2 ½ cups

Egg – 1 plus 2 egg whites

Unrefined sugar – ¼ cup

Vanilla extract – 1 tsp.

Cooking spray

Directions:

- Preheat waffle iron and grease it.
- In a bowl, whisk the dry ingredients. In another bowl, whisk together the wet ingredients. Mix both wet and dry ingredients until just moistened.
- Pour enough batter to cover cooking area. Close the lid.
- Cook until waffle releases from iron.
- Repeat with the remaining batter and serve.

Nutrition:

Calories: 280

Fat: 6g

Carb: 52g

Protein: 14g

8. Blueberry Baked Oatmeal

Preparation Time: 10 minutes

Cooking Time: 30 minutes

Servings: 5

Ingredients:

Cooking spray

Unsweetened soy, rice, or almond milk – 1 cup

Whole egg – 1, plus 2 egg whites

Unsweetened applesauce – ½ cup

Pure maple syrup – 2 Tbsp.

Vanilla extract – ½ tsp.

Baking powder – 1 tsp.

Ground cinnamon – 1 tsp.

Freshly grated nutmeg – 1 pinch

Sea salt – 1 pinch

Old-fashioned rolled oats – 2 ½ cups

Oat bran – ¼ cup

Chopped pecans – ½ cup

Frozen or fresh blueberries – 1 ½ cups, divided

Directions:

- Preheat the oven to 350F.
- Coat a 3-quart casserole dish with cooking spray.
- Whisk together egg, egg whites, milk, applesauce, maple syrup, vanilla, baking powder, cinnamon, sea salt, and nutmeg.
- Mix in oat bran, oats, and pecans.
- Gently fold in half of the blueberries. Scatter remaining blueberries across the bottom of the casserole dish.
- Scrape oatmeal mixture into a casserole dish and bake uncovered for 35 to 40 minutes or until golden brown around the edges.

Nutrition:

Calories: 363

Fat: 10g

Carb: 60g

Protein: 13g

9. French Toast with Strawberries

Preparation Time: 20 minutes

Cooking Time: 7 minutes

Servings: 6

Ingredients:

Firm tofu – 1 (12 oz.) package

Unsweetened soy, rice or almond milk – ½ cup

Pure maple syrup – 2 tsp.

Pure vanilla extract – 1 tsp.

Almond extract – ½ tsp.

Ground cinnamon – ½ tsp.

Pinch sea salt

Coconut oil – 2 Tbsp.

Whole grain bread – 6 slices

Sliced fresh strawberries – 1 ½ cups

Sliced almonds – 6 Tbsp.

Directions:

- To a blender, add the batter and blend until combined well. Pour into a bowl.
- Heat a skillet then grease with oil.

- Dip a slice of bread in batter, then turn it over and dip again to soak completely.
- Place on the griddle and repeat until the griddle is covered with battered bread.
- Sauté bread until the griddle is covered with battered bread.
- Sauté bread until cooked through and browned, 2 to 3 minutes per side.
- Top bread slices with sliced strawberries and almonds and serve.

Nutrition:

Calories: 213

Fat: 11g

Carb: 16g

Protein: 9g

10. Dark and Addictive Bran Muffins

Preparation Time: 25 minutes

Cooking Time: 20 minutes

Servings: 15

Ingredients:

Cooking spray

Boiling water – 1 cup

Wheat bran – 1 cup

Wet ingredients

Coconut oil – 2 Tbsp. melted

Unrefined sugar – ¼ cup

Unsulfured blackstrap molasses

Unsweetened applesauce – ½ cup

Soy, rice or almond milk – 1 cup

Plain soy yogurt – 1 cup

Orange zest – 1 Tbsp.

Dry ingredients

Whole wheat flour – 2 ½ cups

Whole grain soy flour – 2 Tbsp.

Flax meal – 2 Tbsp.

Baking soda – 2 ½ tsp.

Sea salt – ¼ tsp.

All-natural, whole-grain bran flake cereal – 2 cups

Flaxseed for garnish

Directions:

- Keep the oven rack in the center.
- Preheat to 400F.
- Prepare a muffin tin by lining with cooking spray.
- Pour boiling water over bran and set aside.
- Whisk together wet ingredients until combined well.
- In a bowl, whisk together dry ingredients until combined well. Add wet ingredients and mix. Add bran flake cereal and bran and water mixture, stir to combine.
- Divide batter among 15 muffin cups and sprinkle the tops with flaxseeds. Bake for 20 minutes.
- Remove from the oven, cool and serve.

Nutrition:

Calories: 163

Fat: 3g

Carb: 33g

Protein: 3g

Lunch Recipes

11. Rainbow Buddha Bowls

Preparation Time: 10 minutes

Cooking Time: 10 minutes

Servings: 4

Ingredients:

3 cups cooked quinoa

2 cups carrots, shredded or shaved

1½ cups red cabbage, shredded

1½ cups cucumber slices

1 cup fresh spinach

1 red bell pepper, sliced or diced

6 radishes, thinly sliced

1 avocado, sliced

1 cup fresh corn (or frozen and thawed)

¼ cup raw sunflower seeds

Golden Tahini Sauce

Directions:

- Divide the cooked quinoa between 4 bowls.
- Divide the carrots, cabbage, cucumber, spinach, bell pepper, radishes, avocado, corn, and sunflower seeds and place on top of the quinoa in each bowl.

- Drizzle with golden tahini sauce before serving.

Nutrition:

Calories: 489

Total Fat: 24g

Saturated Fat: 3g

Cholesterol: 0mg

Carbohydrates: 60g

Fiber: 13g

Sodium: 505mg

Protein: 15g

12. Sesame Peanut Noodles

Preparation Time: 5 minutes

Cooking Time: 10 minutes

Servings: 4

Ingredients:

12 ounces noodles of choice (ramen, rice, or spaghetti)

5 tablespoons no-salt- and no-sugar-added peanut butter

3 tablespoons coconut aminos or soy sauce

2 tablespoons coconut oil

1½ tablespoons toasted sesame oil

2½ teaspoons maple syrup

¼ teaspoon sea salt

2 teaspoons sesame seeds, for garnish

Directions:

- Cook the noodles according to the package directions.
- In a large bowl, combine the peanut butter, coconut aminos, coconut oil, toasted sesame oil, maple syrup, and salt. Whisk until smooth.
- Toss with the cooked noodles.
- Sprinkle with the sesame seeds before serving.

Nutrition:

Calories: 570

Total Fat: 24g

Saturated Fat: 9g

Cholesterol: 0mg

Carbohydrates: 78g

Fiber: 3g

Sodium: 509mg

Protein: 10g

13. Chickpea Caesar Pitas

Preparation Time: 10 minutes

Cooking Time: 10 minutes

Servings: 4

Ingredients:

FOR THE DRESSING

½ cup mayonnaise

¼ cup vegetarian Parmesan cheese, shredded

2 garlic cloves, grated

1 tablespoon freshly squeezed lemon juice

2 teaspoons Dijon mustard

½ teaspoon freshly ground black pepper

¼ teaspoon sea salt

FOR THE CHICKPEA FILLING

1 romaine heart, chopped

2 cups fresh spinach, chopped

½ cup vegetarian Parmesan cheese

1 tablespoon olive oil

1 (15.5-ounce) can chickpeas, rinsed and drained

2 teaspoons garlic powder

½ teaspoon salt

4 pitas

Directions:

TO MAKE THE DRESSING

- In a large bowl, combine the mayonnaise, Parmesan, garlic, lemon juice, mustard, pepper, and salt and whisk until smooth.
- Set aside.

TO MAKE THE CHICKPEA FILLING

- In a large bowl, combine the chopped romaine, spinach, and Parmesan. Set aside.
  Heat the olive oil in a skillet over medium-high heat. Add the chickpeas and cook for 3 minutes, tossing frequently.
- Add the garlic powder and salt to the chickpeas. Toss to coat, then cook 3 minutes longer, or until crispy and golden.
- Add the chickpeas to the bowl with the dressing and toss to coat. Divide the salad among the pitas to serve.

Nutrition:

Calories: 529

Total Fat: 30g

Saturated Fat: 7g

Cholesterol: 12mg

Carbohydrates: 56g

Fiber: 6g

Sodium: 1,331mg

Protein: 11g

14. White Bean Pasta Salad

Preparation Time: 15 minutes

Cooking Time: 45 minutes

Servings: 4

Ingredients:

FOR THE DRESSING

4 tablespoons freshly squeezed lemon juice

4 tablespoons olive oil

1 tablespoon stone-ground mustard

½ teaspoon sea salt

¼ teaspoon freshly ground black pepper

FOR THE PASTA

8 ounces fusilli pasta

1 (29-ounce) can cannellini beans, rinsed and drained

½ cup red onion, thinly sliced

¼ cup chopped fresh basil

4 garlic cloves, minced

2 tablespoons finely chopped sun-dried tomatoes

Directions:

TO MAKE THE DRESSING

- In a small bowl, combine the lemon juice, olive oil, mustard, salt, and pepper.
- Whisk with a fork until smooth and set aside.

TO MAKE THE PASTA

- Make the pasta according to the package directions.
- Drain, rinse with cold water, and set aside.
- In a large bowl, combine the cannellini beans, red onion, basil, garlic, and sun-dried tomatoes. Fold into the pasta.
- Pour the dressing over the pasta and toss to combine.
- Cover and refrigerate pasta salad for at least 30 minutes before serving.

Nutrition:

Calories: 532

Total Fat: 16g

Saturated Fat: 2g

Cholesterol: 0mg

Carbohydrates: 78g

Fiber: 11g

Sodium: 415mg

Protein: 19g

15. Open-Faced Pesto Melts

Preparation Time: 5 minutes

Cooking Time: 10 minutes

Servings: 4

Ingredients:

8 slices bread of choice (ciabatta, baguette, or focaccia are great choices)

8 tablespoons mayonnaise

8 tablespoons Cashew Basil Pesto or store bought pesto

4 roasted red peppers, halved lengthwise

8 tomato slices, halved

1 cup fresh spinach leaves

8 tablespoons red onion, diced

16 slices provolone cheese, sliced in half

Directions:

- Preheat the oven to 400°F. Place the bread slices on a baking sheet.
- Slather each bread slice with 1 tablespoon of mayonnaise and 1 tablespoon of pesto.
- Top each bread slice with half a roasted red pepper, 2 tomato slice halves, and a few spinach leaves.

- Sprinkle each with 1 tablespoon of diced red onion, and then top each with 1 provolone slice.
- Bake for 5 minutes. Then turn on the broiler and let broil until the cheese is bubbling, about 2 minutes.
- Serve open-faced.

Nutrition:

Calories: 925

Total Fat: 61g

Saturated Fat: 21g

Cholesterol: 70mg

Carbohydrates: 62g

Fiber: 4g

Sodium: 1,789mg

Protein: 33g

16. Costa Rican–Style Gallo Pinto

Preparation Time: 5 minutes

Cooking Time: 10 minutes

Servings: 4

Ingredients:

2 tablespoons oil (such as avocado oil or sunflower oil)

1 onion, diced

3 garlic cloves, minced

1 (15-ounce) can black beans, liquid included

¼ cup Salsa Lizano or vegetarian Worcestershire sauce

2 cups cooked white rice

2 tablespoons chopped fresh cilantro, plus more for garnish

½ teaspoon sea salt

Directions:

- In a large skillet over medium heat, combine the oil, onion, and garlic. Sauté for 5 minutes.
- Add the beans and Salsa Lizano to the skillet. Stir and cook for 2 minutes.
- Add the cooked rice, chopped cilantro, and salt. Mix well and cook for 3 minutes longer, stirring frequently.
- Garnish with fresh chopped cilantro before serving.

Nutrition:

Calories: 287

Total Fat: 8g

Saturated Fat: 1g

Cholesterol: 0mg

Carbohydrates: 48g

Fiber: 9g

Sodium: 851mg

Protein: 9g

17. Crispy Quinoa Cakes

Preparation Time: 10 minutes

Cooking Time: 25 minutes

Servings: 4

Ingredients:

2 tablespoons olive oil, divided

2 cups cooked quinoa

2 eggs

½ cup vegetarian Parmesan cheese

½ cup panko bread crumbs

¼ cup chopped fresh parsley

4 garlic cloves, minced

1 teaspoon garlic powder

¾ teaspoon sea salt

½ teaspoon cumin seeds

½ teaspoon smoked paprika

Directions:

- Heat 1 tablespoon of olive oil in a large skillet over medium heat.
- In a large bowl, combine the cooked quinoa, eggs, cheese, bread crumbs, parsley, garlic, 1 tablespoon of

olive oil, garlic powder, salt, cumin seeds, and smoked paprika. Mix until well combined.

- Using wet hands, form tablespoon-size balls of the quinoa mixture, then flatten into patties using the palm of your hand.
- Gently place in the greased skillet and cook for about 3 minutes or until crispy and golden.
- Gently flip and cook for 3 minutes longer. Repeat with the remaining patties.

Nutrition:

Calories: 253

Total Fat: 10g

Saturated Fat: 3g

Cholesterol: 82mg

Carbohydrates: 34g

Fiber: 3g

Sodium: 766mg

Protein: 9g

18. Butternut Squash Coconut Curry Soup

Preparation Time: 5 minutes

Cooking Time: 30 minutes

Servings: 4

Ingredients:

2 tablespoons coconut oil

1 medium white or yellow onion, diced

2 tablespoons minced garlic

3 tablespoons curry powder

2 tablespoons granulated sugar

2 teaspoons ground turmeric

1 teaspoon ground ginger

½ teaspoon red chili flakes (optional)

4 cups cubed butternut squash (fresh or frozen)

2 (13.5-ounce) cans full-fat coconut milk

¼ cup chopped fresh cilantro, plus more for garnish

1 (14-ounce) package dried rice noodles

2 teaspoons freshly squeezed lemon juice

Sea salt

Directions:

- In a large pot over medium heat, combine the coconut oil, onion, and garlic. Sauté for 5 minutes.
- Stir in the curry powder, sugar, turmeric, ginger, and red chili flakes (if using). Cook for 2 minutes, stirring constantly.
- Stir in the squash and cook for 1 minute longer.
- Pour in the cans of coconut milk, and then use one can to add 6 cans of water to the pot. Stir in the cilantro.
- Turn the heat to high, bring to a boil, reduce to a simmer, and cook for 10 minutes.
- Stir in the rice noodles, lemon juice, and salt to taste. Turn off the heat. Let sit for 10 minutes or until the noodles are tender.
- Ladle into 4 bowls and garnish with cilantro before serving.

Nutrition:

Calories: 895

Total Fat: 42g

Saturated Fat: 36g

Cholesterol: 0mg

Carbohydrates: 124g

Fiber: 13g

Sodium: 799mg

Protein: 12g

19. Mediterranean-Style Cucumber Salad Wraps

Preparation Time: 10 Minutes

Cooking Time: 10 minutes

Servings: 4

Ingredients:

1 cucumber, peel on, diced

1 bell pepper, chopped

½ cup canned chickpeas, rinsed and drained

1/3 cup crumbled feta cheese

¼ cup chopped fresh parsley

¼ cup chopped olives of choice

¼ red onion, diced

1 batch Mediterranean style vinaigrette

4 large tortillas or flatbread wraps of choice

Directions:

- In a large bowl, combine the cucumber, bell pepper, chickpeas, feta, parsley, olives, and onion. Toss to combine.

- Pour the Mediterranean-style vinaigrette over the salad. Toss to coat.
- Divide the salad between the tortillas and roll to wrap.

Nutrition:

Calories: 486

Total Fat: 29g

Saturated Fat: 8g

Cholesterol: 18mg

Carbohydrates: 49g

Fiber: 4g

Sodium: 1,145mg

Protein: 11g

20. Avocado Pesto Pasta with Crispy Garlic Chickpeas

Preparation Time: 10 minutes

Cooking Time: 15 minutes

Servings: 4

Ingredients:

1 pound dry, gluten-free pasta of choice

1 (15-ounce) can chickpeas, rinsed, drained and patted dry

4 tablespoons olive oil, divided

1½ teaspoons sea salt, plus more to taste

2 ripe avocados, peeled and pit removed

¾ cup packed fresh basil leaves

3 tablespoons freshly squeezed lemon juice

1 garlic clove, minced

1/8 teaspoon freshly ground black pepper

2 teaspoons garlic powder

Directions:

- Cook the pasta according to the package directions. Meanwhile, heat a skillet over medium-high heat.
- Combine the chickpeas, 1 tablespoon of olive oil, and ½ teaspoon of salt in the hot skillet. Give a toss, cover, and

let cook while you prepare the pasta sauce. The chickpeas should take 6 to 9 minutes to cook.

- While the chickpeas are cooking, in a food processor or blender, combine the avocados, basil, lemon juice, 3 tablespoons of olive oil, garlic, 1 teaspoon of salt, and pepper.
- Process until smooth and creamy. Taste and adjust salt if necessary.
- Give the chickpeas another toss; they should begin to turn golden and crispy. Turn off heat and toss with the garlic powder. Let sit and salt to taste.
- When the pasta is tender, drain and then immediately toss with the avocado sauce. Top with the crispy chickpeas before serving.

Nutrition:

Calories: 759

Total Fat: 28g

Saturated Fat: 4g

Cholesterol: 0mg

Carbohydrates: 108g

Fiber: 13g

Sodium: 1,039mg

Protein: 22g

Dinner
Recipes

21. Eggplant Kufta

Preparation Time: 15 minutes

Cooking Time: 30 minutes

Servings: 4

Ingredients:

1 large eggplant, cut into 2-inch cubes

¼ cup olive oil, divided

1 small onion, chopped

½ cup chopped fresh parsley

¼ cup chopped fresh cilantro

2 garlic cloves, minced

1 teaspoon sweet paprika

½ teaspoon ground coriander

¼ teaspoon cayenne pepper

1/8 teaspoon salt, plus more as needed

½ cup coarsely chopped almonds

2 cups bread crumbs

Directions:

- Preheat the broiler.
- In a large bowl, combine the eggplant and 2 table-spoons of olive oil. Toss well to coat. Spread the eggplant on a baking sheet. Broil for about 5 minutes until golden. Remove and let cool.
- Reduce the oven temperature to 400°F.
- Transfer the cooled eggplant to a food processor and purée. Transfer the eggplant purée to a medium bowl.
- In the food processor, combine the onion, parsley, and cilantro. Purée.
- Add this herb mixture to the eggplant, along with the garlic, paprika, coriander, cayenne, salt, almonds, and bread crumbs. Stir until well combined. Taste and season with more salt as needed.
- Moisten your palms with the remaining 2 tablespoons of olive oil. Form the eggplant mixture into 3-inch balls and place them on a baking sheet. You should have about 20 balls.
- Bake for 20 minutes. Flip the balls and bake for 5 minutes more until firm.

Nutrition:

Calories: 478

Total Fat: 24g

Saturated Fat: 3g

Carbohydrates: 56g

Fiber: 10g

Protein: 13g

Sodium: 213mg

22. Bell Pepper and Onion Tart

Preparation Time: 15 minutes

Cooking Time: 40 minutes

Servings: 6

Ingredients:

2 tablespoons olive oil

1 red onion, chopped

All-purpose flour, for dusting

1 refrigerated store bought piecrust

1 cup ricotta

½ cup heavy cream

2 large eggs

¼ cup chopped fresh basil

1/8 teaspoon salt

1/8 teaspoon freshly ground black pepper

2 red bell peppers, seeded and thinly sliced

Directions:

- Preheat the oven to 425°F.
- In a skillet over medium heat, heat the olive oil. Add the red onion and cook for 10 minutes or until softened.

- Dust a work surface with flour and place the crust on it. Let the crust sit for 10 minutes. Transfer the crust, flour-side down, to a 9-inch tart pan. Gently push the crust against the edges.
- Pierce the bottom of the crust in a few places with a fork and bake for 10 minutes. Remove and set aside to cool.
- In a medium bowl, stir together the ricotta, heavy cream, eggs, basil, salt, and pepper. Set aside.
- Spoon the cooked onion onto the baked piecrust. Spoon the cheese mixture over the onion and arrange the red bell peppers over the cheese.
- Bake for about 20 minutes or until the filling is set.

Nutrition:

Calories: 315

Total Fat: 24g

Saturated Fat: 9g

Carbohydrates: 18g

Fiber: 1g

Protein: 9g

Sodium: 268mg

23. Chakchouka

Preparation Time: 10 minutes

Cooking Time: 25 minutes

Servings: 4

Ingredients:

¼ cup olive oil

1 onion, finely chopped

1 cup chopped green bell pepper

2 garlic cloves, minced

3 ripe tomatoes, diced

1 teaspoon paprika

½ teaspoon ground cumin

½ teaspoon red pepper flakes

1/8 teaspoon salt

4 medium eggs

Directions:

- In a large sauté pan or skillet over medium heat, heat the olive oil.
- Add the onion and green bell pepper. Cook for about 8 minutes until the vegetables soften. Add the garlic and cook for 1 minute more.

- In a small bowl, stir together the tomatoes, paprika, cumin, red pepper flakes, and salt until well combined. Add the tomato mixture to the pan, stir, and simmer for 8 minutes.
- Gently crack the eggs on top of the cooked vegetables, being careful not to break the yolks. Cover the pan and cook for 5 minutes or until the egg yolks are firm but not dry.

Nutrition:

Calories: 225

Total Fat: 19g

Saturated Fat: 3g

Carbohydrates: 10g

Fiber: 2g

Protein: 7g

Sodium: 143mg

24. Asparagus and Swiss Quiche

Preparation Time: 20 minutes

Cooking Time: 50 minutes

Servings: 6

Ingredients:

6 cups water

8 ounces asparagus, ends trimmed, cut into 1-inch pieces

2 tablespoons olive oil

4 scallions, white and green parts, chopped

1 (8-inch) store bought unbaked pie shell

2 large eggs

½ cup heavy cream

2 tablespoons chopped fresh tarragon

¼ teaspoon ground nutmeg

1 cup shredded Swiss cheese

Directions:

- Preheat the oven to 400°F.
- In a medium pot over medium-high heat, bring the water to a boil. Drop the asparagus into the boiling water and blanch for 2 minutes. Drain and set aside.

- In a skillet over medium heat, heat the olive oil. Add the scallions and cook for 5 minutes. Add the asparagus and cook for 1 minute.
- Spoon the vegetables into the unbaked pie shell. Set aside.
- In a medium bowl, whisk the eggs. Add the heavy cream, tarragon, and nutmeg. Whisk to combine well.
- Pour the egg mixture over the asparagus. Sprinkle the Swiss cheese over the top.
- Bake for about 40 minutes until firm. Remove from the oven, cool to room temperature, and serve.

Nutrition:

Calories: 319

Total Fat: 26g

Saturated Fat: 10g

Carbohydrates: 15g

Fiber: 1g

Protein: 9g

Sodium: 202mg

25. Spinach and Mushroom Gratin

Preparation Time: 10 minutes

Cooking Time: 40 minutes

Servings: 8

Ingredients:

4 tablespoons butter

1 large onion, chopped

1 pound shiitake mushrooms, coarsely chopped

1 cup heavy cream

1 cup milk

2 tablespoons cornstarch

2 tablespoons cold water

¼ teaspoon grated nutmeg

1/8 teaspoon salt

1/8 teaspoon freshly ground black pepper

1 (16-ounce) package frozen chopped spinach, thawed and squeezed dry

½ cup freshly grated Parmesan cheese

½ cup grated Gruyère cheese

Directions:

- Preheat the oven to 400°F.
- In a heavy-bottomed saucepan over medium heat, melt the butter. Add the onion and cook for 5 minutes. Add the mushrooms and cook for 10 minutes or until browned.
- In a small bowl, whisk the heavy cream and milk.
- In another small bowl, stir together the cornstarch and cold water until the cornstarch dissolves. Add this slurry to the milk mixture and stir to combine.
- Pour the milk mixture over the mushrooms. Stir in the nutmeg, salt, and pepper. Cook for about 5 minutes until the sauce thickens.
- Add the spinach to the sauce. Stir in the Parmesan cheese. Spoon the spinach and mushroom mixture into a gratin baking dish. Sprinkle the Gruyère cheese on top.
- Bake for about 20 minutes until hot and bubbly.

Nutrition:

Calories: 278

Total Fat: 22g

Saturated Fat: 13g

Carbohydrates: 16g

Fiber: 3g

Protein: 9g

Sodium: 368mg

26. Cherry Tomato, Olive, And Sourdough Gratin

Preparation Time: 20 minutes

Cooking Time: 45 minutes

Servings: 6

Ingredients:

1 sourdough loaf, cut into 1-inch cubes (about 6 cups)

1 cup pitted cured black olives, halved lengthwise, divided

1 (12-ounce) can diced tomatoes

6 scallions, white and green parts, chopped

1 cup chopped fresh basil

1/8 teaspoon salt, plus more as needed

1/8 teaspoon freshly ground black pepper, plus more as needed

1 cup shredded Manchego cheese

4 cups cherry tomatoes, halved lengthwise

Directions:

- Preheat the oven to 375°F.
- Place the bread in a large bowl. Chop half the olives and add them to the bread, along with the diced tomatoes, scallions, basil, salt, and pepper. Stir until well

combined. Taste and season with more salt and pepper, as needed.

- Spoon the mixture into a 9-by-13-inch baking dish. Top the bread mixture with the Manchego cheese. Arrange the cherry tomatoes and the remaining olives on top of the cheese. Cover the dish with aluminum foil.
- Bake for 20 minutes. Remove the foil and bake for 15 minutes more until the cheese is melted and the edges of the bread are golden. Let rest for 10 minutes before serving.

Nutrition:

Calories: 324

Total Fat: 11g

Saturated Fat: 4g

Carbohydrates: 42g

Fiber: 3g

Protein: 13g

Sodium: 536mg

27. Ratatouille

Preparation Time: 20 minutes

Cooking Time: 35 minutes

Servings: 4

Ingredients:

¼ cup olive oil

1 onion, chopped

4 garlic cloves, crushed

1 large eggplant, cut into 1-inch cubes

1 zucchini, cut into 1-inch cubes

1 red bell pepper, seeded and chopped

1/8 teaspoon salt, plus more as needed

3 tomatoes, chopped

1 tablespoon dried oregano

1 teaspoon dried thyme

¼ cup chopped fresh basil

Directions:

- In a heavy-bottomed skillet over medium heat, heat the olive oil.
- Add the onion and cook for 5 minutes or until soft. Add the garlic and cook for 2 minutes.

- Add the eggplant and cook for 10 minutes, stirring often.
- Stir in the zucchini, red bell pepper, and salt. Cook for 5 minutes.
- Stir in the tomatoes, oregano, thyme, and basil. Cook for 10 minutes. Taste and season with more salt, as needed.

Nutrition:

Calories: 191

Total Fat: 13g

Saturated Fat: 2g

Carbohydrates: 19g

Fiber: 7g

Protein: 4g

Sodium: 88mg

28. French Bean Stew

Preparation Time: 10 minutes

Cooking Time: 40 minutes

Servings: 4

Ingredients:

¼ cup olive oil

1 onion, chopped

1 pound French green beans, trimmed and cut into 2-inch pieces

4 ripe tomatoes, seeded and diced, or 1 (28-ounce) can diced tomatoes, undrained

4 garlic cloves, minced

1/8 teaspoon salt

1/8 teaspoon freshly ground black pepper

2 tablespoons tomato paste

2 cups vegetable broth

Directions:

- In a soup pot over medium heat, heat the olive oil. Add the onion and cook for 5 minutes, stirring often, until softened.

- Add the green beans, cover the pot, and cook for 10 minutes, stirring often. If necessary, add 2 tablespoons of water to prevent the beans from sticking.
- Stir in the tomatoes and their juices, garlic, salt, and pepper. Cook for 10 minutes.
- In a medium bowl, whisk the tomato paste and vegetable broth until completely combined. Pour the broth into the pot. Bring the stew to a boil. Cover the pot and simmer for 15 minutes.
- Taste and season with more salt and pepper as needed before serving.

Nutrition:

Calories: 207

Total Fat: 14g

Saturated Fat: 2g

Carbohydrates: 18g

Fiber: 6g

Protein: 6g

Sodium: 378mg

29. Eggplant And Lentil Tagine

Preparation Time: 15 minutes

Cooking Time: 40 minutes

Servings: 6

Ingredients:

1 eggplant, cut into 1-inch cubes

½ cup olive oil, divided

2 onions, thinly sliced

1 cup chopped fresh cilantro

3 tablespoons tomato paste

2 tablespoons Harissa, or store bought

2 teaspoons ground coriander

1 teaspoon ground cumin

1-pound dried brown lentils, rinsed and picked over for debris

8 cups water

1/8 teaspoon salt, plus more as needed

1/8 teaspoon freshly ground black pepper, plus more as needed

2 cups fresh baby spinach

1 cup diced dried apricots

½ cup freshly squeezed lemon juice

2 tablespoons chopped preserved lemons, or store bought

Directions:

- Preheat the broiler.
- In a medium bowl, toss the eggplant with 2 tablespoons of olive oil to coat. Transfer to a baking sheet and broil for about 5 minutes until golden. Remove and set aside.
- In a large soup pot over medium heat, heat the remaining 6 tablespoons of olive oil.
- Add the onions and cook for about 8 minutes until golden. Add the cilantro and cook for 1 minute. Using a slotted spoon, transfer half the onion mixture to a bowl and set aside.
- Add the tomato paste, harissa, coriander, and cumin to the pot. Stir to combine and cook for 1 minute.
- Stir in the lentils, water, salt, and pepper. Taste and season with more salt and pepper, as needed. Increase the heat to bring the mixture to a boil.
- Reduce the heat to medium and cook for about 15 minutes or until the lentils are tender.
- Stir in the eggplant, spinach, apricots, lemon juice, and preserved lemons. Cook for 10 minutes more.
- Spoon the tagine onto a platter and top with the remaining cooked onion and cilantro mixture.

Nutrition:

Calories: 526

Total Fat: 18g

Saturated Fat: 3g

Carbohydrates: 72g

Fiber: 29g

Protein: 23g

Sodium: 82mg

30. Roasted Cauliflower Tagine

Preparation Time: 15 minutes

Cooking Time: 35 minutes

Servings: 6

Ingredients:

2 cauliflower heads, cut into florets

½ cup olive oil, divided

½ cup chopped fresh cilantro

1 onion, chopped

6 garlic cloves, peeled

1 teaspoon ground coriander

1 (32-ounce) can diced tomatoes

1 tablespoon tomato paste

6 cups water

1/8 teaspoon salt, plus more as needed

1/8 teaspoon freshly ground black pepper, plus more as needed

2 large russet potatoes, peeled and cut into 1-inch cubes

1 (15-ounce) can chickpeas, drained and rinsed

¼ cup chopped Preserved Lemons, or store bought

Directions:

- Preheat the broiler.
- In a medium bowl, toss the cauliflower and 2 table-spoons of olive oil until well coated. Transfer the florets to a baking sheet and broil for about 5 minutes until golden. Remove and set aside.
- In a small skillet over medium heat, heat 2 tablespoons of olive oil. Add the cilantro and sear for a few seconds. Set aside.
- In a heavy-bottomed pot over medium heat, heat the remaining 4 tablespoons of olive oil. Add the onion and sauté for 2 to 3 minutes until golden. Stir in the garlic and coriander. Cook for 1 minute more.
- Stir in the tomatoes, tomato paste, water, salt, and pepper until well combined. Taste and season with more salt and pepper, as needed. Increase the heat to medium-high and bring to a boil. Turn the heat to low and simmer for 5 minutes.
- Stir in the potatoes, increase the heat to high, and return the mixture to a boil. Reduce the heat to medium and cook for about 10 minutes until the potatoes are fork-tender but not overcooked.
- Add the chickpeas, roasted cauliflower, and cilantro. Stir gently and cook over low heat for 10 minutes to warm through. Sprinkle with the preserved lemons and serve.

Nutrition:

Calories: 378

Total Fat: 19g

Saturated Fat: 3g

Carbohydrates: 48g

Fiber: 13g

Protein: 11g

Sodium: 126mg

Side Recipes

31. Nutmeg Green Beans

Preparation Time: 10 minutes

Cooking Time: 30 minutes

Servings: 4

Ingredients:

2 tablespoons olive oil

½ cup coconut cream

1-pound green beans, trimmed and halved

1 teaspoon nutmeg, ground

A pinch of salt and cayenne pepper

½ teaspoon onion powder

½ teaspoon garlic powder

2 tablespoons parsley, chopped

Directions:

- Heat a pan with the oil over medium heat, add the green beans, nutmeg and the other ingredients, toss, cook for 30 minutes.
- Divide the mix between plates and serve.

Nutrition:

Calories 100

Fat 13g

Fiber 2.3g

Carbs 5.1g

Protein 2g

32. Peppers and Celery Sauté

Preparation Time: 10 minutes

Cooking Time: 15 minutes

Servings: 4

Ingredients:

1 red bell pepper, cut into medium chunks

1 green bell pepper, cut into medium chunks

1 celery stalk, chopped

2 scallions, chopped

2 tablespoons olive oil

Salt and black pepper to taste

1 tablespoons parsley, chopped

1 teaspoon cumin, ground

2 garlic cloves, minced

Directions:

- Heat a pan with the oil over medium heat, add the scallions, garlic and cumin and sauté for 5 minutes.
- Add the peppers, celery and the other ingredients, toss, cook over medium heat for 10 minutes more, divide between plates and serve.

Nutrition:

Calories 87

Fat 2.4g

Fiber 3g

Carbs 5g

Protein 4g

33. Oregano Zucchinis and Broccoli

Preparation Time: 10 minutes

Cooking Time: 20 minutes

Servings: 4

Ingredients:

1-pound zucchinis, sliced

1 cup broccoli florets

Salt and black pepper to taste

2 tablespoons avocado oil

2 tablespoons chili powder

½ teaspoon oregano, dried

1 and ½ tablespoons coriander, chopped

Directions:

- Heat a pan with the oil over medium heat, add the zucchinis, broccoli and the other ingredients, toss, cook over medium heat for 20 minutes.
- Divide between plates and serve as a side dish.

Nutrition:

Calories 140

Fat 2g

Fiber 1g

Carbs 1g

Protein 6g

34. Spinach Mash

Preparation Time: 10 minutes

Cooking Time: 15 minutes

Servings: 4

Ingredients:

1 pound spinach leaves

3 scallions, chopped

2 garlic cloves, minced

¼ cup coconut cream

2 tablespoons olive oil

Salt and black pepper to taste

½ tablespoon chives, chopped

Directions:

- Heat a pan with the oil over medium heat, add the scallions and the garlic and sauté for 2 minutes.
- Add the spinach and the other ingredients except the chives, toss, cook over medium heat for 13 minutes, blend using an immersion blender.
- Divide between plates, sprinkle the chives on top and serve.

Nutrition:

Calories 190

Fat 16g

Fiber 7g

Carbs 3g

Protein 5g

35. Jalapeno Zucchinis Mix

Preparation Time: 10 minutes

Cooking Time: 30 minutes

Servings: 4

Ingredients:

1-pound zucchinis, sliced

¼ cup green onions, chopped

½ cup cashew cheese, shredded

1 cup coconut cream

2 jalapenos, chopped

Salt and black pepper to taste

2 tablespoons chives, chopped

Directions:

- In a baking dish, combine the zucchinis with the onions and the other ingredients, toss, bake at 390 degrees F for 30 minutes.
- Divide between plates and serve.

Nutrition:

Calories 120

Fat 4.2g

Fiber 2.3g

Carbs 3g

Protein 6g

36. Coconut and Tomatoes Mix

Preparation Time: 5 minutes

Cooking Time: 12 minutes

Servings: 4

Ingredients:

1-pound tomatoes, cut into wedges

1 cup coconut, unsweetened and shredded

2 tablespoons coconut oil, melted

1 tablespoon chives, chopped

1 teaspoon coriander, ground

1 teaspoon fennel seeds

Salt and black pepper to taste

Directions:

- Heat a pan with the oil over medium heat, add the coriander and fennel seeds and cook for 2 minutes.
- Add the tomatoes and the other ingredients, toss, cook over medium heat for 10 minutes, divide between plates and serve.

Nutrition:

Calories 152

Fat 13.8g

Fiber 3.4g

Carbs 7.7g

Protein 1.8g

37. Mushroom Rice

Preparation Time: 10 minutes

Cooking Time: 20 minutes

Servings: 4

Ingredients:

2 tablespoons olive oil

1 cup mushrooms, sliced

2 cups cauliflower rice

2 tablespoons lime juice

2 tablespoons almonds, sliced

1 cup veggie stock

Salt and black pepper to taste

½ teaspoon garlic powder

1 tablespoon parsley, chopped

Directions:

- Heat a pan with the oil over medium heat, add the mushrooms and the almonds and sauté for 5 minutes.
- Add the cauliflower rice and the other ingredients, toss, cook over medium heat for 15 minutes more.
- Divide between plates and serve.

Nutrition:

Calories 124

Fat 2.4g

Fiber 1.5g

Carbs 2g

Protein 1.2g

38. Cucumber and Cauliflower Mix

Preparation Time: 10 minutes

Cooking Time: 12 minutes

Servings: 4

Ingredients:

1 cucumber, cubed

1 pound cauliflower florets

1 spring onion, chopped

2 tablespoons avocado oil

1 tablespoon balsamic vinegar

¼ teaspoon red pepper flakes

Salt and black pepper to taste

1 tablespoon thyme, chopped

Directions:

- Heat a pan with the oil over medium heat, add the spring onions and the pepper flakes and sauté for 2 minutes.
- Add the cucumber and the other ingredients, toss, cook over medium heat for 10 minutes more.
- Divide between plates and serve.

Nutrition:

Calories 53

Fat 1.2g

Fiber 3.9g

Carbs 9.9g

Protein 3g

39. Mushroom and Spinach Mix

Preparation Time: 10 minutes

Cooking Time: 15 minutes

Servings: 4

Ingredients:

1 cup white mushrooms, sliced

3 cups baby spinach

2 tablespoons olive oil

Salt and black pepper to taste

2 tablespoons garlic, minced

2 tablespoons pine nuts, toasted

1 tablespoon walnuts, chopped

Directions:

- Heat a pan with the oil over medium heat, add the garlic, pine nuts and the walnuts and cook for 5 minutes.
- Add the mushrooms and the other ingredients, toss, cook over medium heat for 10 minutes, divide between plates and serve.

Nutrition:

Calories 116

Fat 11.3g

Fiber 1.1g

Carbs 3.5g

Protein 2.5g

40. Garlic Cauliflower Rice

Preparation Time: 10 minutes

Cooking Time: 20 minutes

Servings: 4

Ingredients:

2 cups cauliflower rice

2 tablespoons almonds, chopped

1 tablespoon olive oil

2 green onions, chopped

4 garlic cloves, minced

3 tablespoons chives, chopped

½ cup vegetable stock

Directions:

- Heat a pan with the oil over medium heat, add the garlic and green onions and sauté for 5 minutes.
- Add the cauliflower rice and the other ingredients, toss, cook over medium heat for 15 minutes, divide between plates and serve.

Nutrition:

Calories 142

Fat 6.1g

Fiber 1.2g

Carbs 3g

Protein 1.2g

Dessert

Recipes

41. Cinnamon Ice Cream

Preparation Time: 30 minutes

Cooking Time: 10 minutes

Servings: 6

Ingredients:

Regular black tea – 4 bags

Full fat coconut milk – 2 cans (28 ounces)

Honey – ¾ cup

Pure vanilla extract – 1 tsp.

Ground ginger – ¾ tsp.

Cinnamon – ¾ tsp.

Cardamom – ¼ tsp.

Cloves – ¼ tsp.

Allspice – ¼ tsp.

Fine-grain Sea salt – 1 pinch

Arrowroot starch – 1 ½ tsp. whisked with a few Tbsp. of the coconut milk mixture

Directions:

- In a liquid measuring cup, add the tea bags, and pour one cup boiling water. Steep for 4 minutes, then remove the tea bags.

- Shake the coconut milk cans before opening. In a Dutch oven, whisk together the honey, vanilla, tea, coconut milk, spices, and salt and mix well.
- Heat the mixture over medium heat. Whisk the arrowroot starch with a few Tbsp. of the coconut milk mixture in a small bowl until mixed well.
- Add the arrowroot mixture to the warm coconut milk mixture and bring the mixture to a gentle boil. Stir constantly for 1 minute.
- Remove and cool. Then chill in the refrigerator. Also, place the ice cream container to chill.
- With a spoon, scoop off the thickened top layer. Whisk the chilled mixture for 1 last time, then pour into your ice cream maker.
- Freeze according to the manufacturer's instructions. Then place in the chilled container and freeze for a few hours in the freezer.

Nutrition:

Calories: 356

Fat: 24.1g

Carb: 38.8g

Protein: 2.6g

42. Caramel-Apple Pudding Cake

Preparation Time: 10 minutes

Cooking Time: 35 minutes

Servings: 12

Ingredients:

Jonathan or Granny Smith apples – 2 medium (prepared and thinly sliced)

Lemon juice – 3 Tbsp.

Ground cinnamon – ½ tsp.

Ground nutmeg – 1/8 tsp.

Raisins – ¼ cup

All-purpose flour – 1 cup

Brown sugar – ¾ cup, packed

Baking powder – 1 tsp.

Baking soda – ¼ tsp.

Milk – ½ cup

Butter – 2 Tbsp. melted

Vanilla – 1 tsp.

Chopped walnuts or pecans – ½ cup

Caramel ice cream topping – ¾ cup

Water – ½ cup

Butter – 1 Tbsp.

Directions:

Preheat the oven to 350F.

- In the bottom of a greased 2-quart square baking dish arrange apple slices. Sprinkle with nutmeg, cinnamon and lemon juice. Top with raisins and set aside.
- In a bowl, combine brown sugar, flour, baking soda, and baking powder. Add vanilla, 2 Tbsp. melted butter and milk. Mix well and stir in nuts. Spread batter evenly over apple mixture.
- In a small saucepan, combine 1 Tbsp. butter, water, and caramel topping. Bring to a boil. Into the baking dish pour the caramel mixture (over the batter).
- Bake in the oven until set in the center, about 35 minutes.
- Serve in individual dessert dishes. Spoon apple-caramel mixture over each portion.

Nutrition:

Calories: 223

Fat: 6g

Carb: 42g

Protein: 2g

43. Caramel-Pecan French Silk Pie

Preparation Time: 10 minutes

Cooking Time: 15 minutes

Servings: 8

Ingredients:

Baked pastry shell – 1

Whipping cream – 1 cup

Semisweet chocolate pieces– 1 cup

Butter – 1/3 cup

Sugar – 1/3 cup

Egg yolks – 2, lightly beaten

Whipping cream or cream de cacao – 3 Tbsp.

Caramel ice cream topping – 1 (12 ¼ ounce) jar

Coarsely chopped – ¾ cup, toasted almonds or pecans

Whipped cream – 1 cup

Chocolate curls

Directions:

- Prepare baked pastry shell. Set aside
- Combine the sugar, butter, chocolate pieces, and 1 cup whipping cream in a heavy medium saucepan.

- Cook over low heat for 10 minutes or until chocolate is melted. Stirring constantly. Remove from the heat.
- Bit-by-bit stir half of the hot mixture into the beaten egg yolks.
- Return egg mixture to chocolate mixture in the pan.
- Cook on medium-low for 5 minutes or until mixture starts to bubble and slightly thickened. Remove from the heat.
- Stir in the whipping cream or the crème de cacao. In a bowl of ice water, place the saucepan for 20 minutes (stir occasionally) or until the mixture becomes hard to stir. Transfer to a bowl.
- Beat cooled chocolate mixture with a hand mixer on high speed until light and fluffy, about 2 to 3 minutes.
- In the bottom of the baked pastry shell, spread caramel ice cream topping.
- Sprinkle with pecans. Gently spread filling into pie shell.
- Cover and refrigerate pie overnight.
- Top with whipped cream, garnish with chocolate nuts and serve.

Nutrition:

Calories: 725

Fat: 47g

Carb: 72g

Protein: 6g

44. Peach Caramel Blondie Bars

Preparation Time: 10 minutes

Cooking Time: 20 minutes

Servings: 16

Ingredients:

All-purpose flour – ¾ cup

Baking powder – ½ tsp.

Salt – ¼ tsp.

Butter – ¼, cup, softened

Sugar – 2/3 cup

Egg – 1

White baking chocolate – 2 ounces, chopped

Caramel-flavored ice cream topping – ½ cup

Fresh peaches – 2 small, prepared and sliced

Pistachio nuts – 1/3 cup, coarsely chopped

Directions:

- Preheat the oven to 325F. Line and grease a (9x9x2-inch) baking (cover the edges of the pan).
- For the crust, combine baking powder, flour, and salt in a bowl. In another bowl, beat butter with a hand mixer speed for 30 seconds (on medium speed).

- Add sugar and beat for 5 minutes. Scape the sides as needed.
- Add egg and continue to beat.
- Add the flour mixture slowly and beat on until combined (on low speed).
- Spread the batter evenly in the prepared pan.
- Bake until feels nearly firm in the center and crust is lightly browned, about 20 minutes. Cool slightly on wire rack.
- Melt white chocolate. Spread evenly over the crust. Chill briefly until set.
- Remove the uncut bars from the pan. Spread with dulce de leche.
- Cut into bars. Sprinkle with pistachios and top with peaches. Serve.

Nutrition:

Calories: 155

Fat: 6g

Carb: 23g

Protein: 3g

45. Strawberry Greek Frozen Yogurt

Preparation Time: 10 minutes

Cooking Time: 0 minutes

Servings: 16

Ingredients:

Plan Greek low-fat yogurt – 3 cups

Sugar – 1 cup

Freshly squeezed lemon juice – ¼ cup

Vanilla – 2 tsp.

Salt – 1/8 tsp.

Sliced strawberries – 1 cup

Directions:

- Combine the lemon juice, sugar, yogurt, vanilla and salt in a bowl. Whisk until smooth.
- In an ice cream maker, freeze the mixture according to the instructions. Add the strawberries at the last minute.
- Then freeze a few hours before serving.
- Let stand at room temperature for 10 minutes and serve.

Nutrition:

Calories: 86

Fat: 1g

Carb: 16g

Protein: 4g

46. Greek Almond Shortbread Cookies

Preparation Time: 10 minutes

Cooking Time: 15 minutes

Servings: 8

Ingredients:

Butter – 1 ½ cup, softened

Powdered sugar – 1 cup

Egg yolks – 2

Brandy or orange juice – 2 Tbsp.

Vanilla – 2 tsp.

Cake flour – 3 ½ cups

Blanched almonds – 1 cup, lightly toasted and finely ground

Powdered sugar

Rose flower water – 2 Tbsp.

Directions:

- Beat butter in a bowl with a hand mixer on high speed for 30 seconds.
- Add 1 cup powdered sugar and beat until mixture is light in color and fluffy. Beat in brandy, egg yolks, and vanilla until combined.
- Stir in almonds and flour with a wooden spoon. Cover and chill until dough is easy to handle, about 1 hour.

- Preheat the oven to 325F. Shape dough small balls and place on an ungreased cookie sheet (2-inches apart). Flatten the balls to ¼-inch thickness with the bottom of a glass (dipped in powdered sugar).
- Bake in the preheated oven until set, about 12 to 14 minutes. Transfer cookies to a wire rack. Lightly brush the cookies with rose water while still warm. Sprinkle with powdered sugar.
- Cool on wire rack.

Nutrition:

Calories: 78

Fat: 4.7g

Carb: 8.3g

Protein: 1g

47. Sweet Ricotta and Strawberry Parfaits

Preparation Time: 10 minutes

Cooking Time: 0 minutes

Servings: 6

Ingredients:

Fresh strawberries – 1 pound, prepared and quartered

Sugar – 1 tsp.

Snipped fresh mint – 1 Tbsp.

Part-skim ricotta cheese – 1 (15-ounce) cartoon

Light agave nectar – 3 Tbsp.

Vanilla – ½ tsp.

Finely shredded lemon peel – ¼ tsp.

Fresh mint

Directions:

- Combine sugar, strawberries, and 1 Tbsp. mint in a bowl. Stir gently and combine. Let stand until berries soften and release their juices, about 10 minutes.
- In another bowl, combine lemon peel, vanilla, agave nectar, and ricotta. Beat with a hand mixer for 2 minutes on medium speed.
- Assemble in parfait glasses by repeating layers of ricotta mixture and strawberry mixture.

- Garnish with mint and serve.

Nutrition:

Calories: 157

Fat: 6g

Carb: 18g

Protein: 9g

48. Almond Icebox Rounds

Preparation Time: 10 minutes

Cooking Time: 15 minutes

Servings: 6

Ingredients:

Butter – 1 cup, softened

Cream cheese – 1 (3 ounce) package, softened

Sugar – 2/3 cup

Salt – ½ tsp.

Vanilla – ½ tsp.

Almond extract – ¼ tsp.

All-purpose flour – 2 cups

Slivered almonds – ¾ cup, toasted and chopped

Sliced almonds – 2/3 cup, chopped

Directions:

- Combine the butter and cream cheese. Use a hand mixer to beat for 30 seconds. Add almond extract, vanilla, salt, and sugar. Beat until combined.
- Beat in as much as flour as you can with the mixer. Stir in remaining flour with a wooden spoon and ¾ cup toasted almonds.

- Divide dough in half and shape each half into an 8-inch roll.
- In 2/3 cup almonds roll each roll of dough.
- Wrap each roll in plastic or waxed rap. Chill until firm enough to slice, about 6 hours.
- Preheat the oven to 350F.
- Line a cookie sheet with parchment paper and cut rolls into ¼ inch slices.
- On the prepared baking cookie sheet, place slices 1-inch apart.
- Bake for 12 to 14 minutes.
- Cool on a wire rack.

Nutrition:

Calories: 74

Fat: 5.2g

Carb: 6.1g

Protein: 1.2g

49. Bread Pudding with Rum Sauce

Preparation Time: 10 minutes

Cooking Time: 50 minutes

Servings: 8

Ingredients:

Eggs – 4, beaten

Milk – 2 ¼ cups

Sugar – ½ cup

Vanilla – 1 Tbsp.

Ground cinnamon – ½ tsp.

Cinnamon rolls – 4 cups, cut into ¼ inch and toasted

Dried cranberries, cherries or raisins – 1/3 cup

Whipped cream

Directions:

- Beat together milk, cinnamon, vanilla, sugar, and eggs in a bowl.
- Toss together dried fruit and cinnamon roll pieces in an ungreased 2-quart square baking dish. Pour egg mixture evenly over roll mixture. Press with a spoon to coat all the roll pieces.
- Bake, uncovered in a 350F oven until puffed, about 40 to 45 minutes. Cool slightly.

- To make the sauce: combine corn syrup, butter, whipping cream, and brown sugar in a heavy saucepan. Bring to a boil over medium-high heat. Whisk occasionally.
- Lower heat and gently boil for 3 minutes. Remove from the heat and stir in salt, vanilla, and rum.
- Serve with whipped cream and caramel sauce.

Nutrition:

Calories: 479

Fat: 29.3g

Carb: 46.6g

Protein: 7.7g

50. Flourless Brownies

Preparation Time: 10 minutes

Cooking Time: 20 minutes

Servings: 6

Ingredients:

Overripe bananas – 3 medium

Smooth almond butter – ½ cup

Cocoa powder – ¼ cup

Directions:

- Preheat the oven to 350F. Grease a small cake pans and set aside.
- Melt the nut butter in the microwave.
- In a mixing bowl, add the cocoa powder, nut butter, and banana. Mix really well.
- Pour the mixture into the greased pan.
- Bake in the oven for 20 minutes.
- Remove from the oven, cool completely. Slice and serve.

Nutrition:

Calories: 69

Fat: 1.4g

Carb: 15.7g

Protein: 1.6g

Conclusion

A vegetarian diet consists of a plant-based diet that excludes meat and any other animal products. It is one of the most popular diets in the world, with an annual meat consumption rate of only 10%. Most vegetarians are vegans, who exclude not only meat but also dairy and eggs.

The earliest forms of this diet were in India where people made commitments to go vegan for religious purposes or as part of their ascetic practices during which they would grow their own food, eat fruit from trees, milk from cows (or goats), honey from bees - all so that they could follow strict vegetarian diets while still consuming some kind of food product.

As this is the end of this book, I would like to share with you some benefits of being a vegetarian to keep you inspired:

1. More lean muscle mass

Vegetables and fruits are loaded with protein: beans, nuts, seeds, and whole grains all packed with a great amount of lean muscle mass building protein. While some vegetarians who eat meat will choose to eat chicken or fish to get the protein they need, many do not eat meat at all.

2. Lower heart disease risk

The vegetarian diet includes high amounts of fruits and vegetables in the daily diet as well as eating healthy fats like nuts, seeds and avocados. Red meat is a major source of saturated fat which has been linked to an increase in heart disease risk. Studies show that vegetarians have a significantly lower heart disease risk.

3. Lower cholesterol and disease risk

Studies show that vegetarians have an average blood cholesterol level only about half as high as the typical American's level. In fact, a vegetarian diet was shown to lower cholesterol levels more effectively than the whole grain and low-fat diets recommended by the American Heart Association. Relatively speaking, a well-planned vegetarian diet can help lower your LDL (bad) cholesterol while increasing your HDL (good) cholesterol levels for improved cardiovascular health.

4. Lowers risk of cancer

Protein and iron are critical for promoting healthy body cells, cell growth and cancer prevention by keeping inflammation down and cellular communication maintained. If you are not getting enough protein and iron, your body may be more susceptible to cancerous cell growth.

5. Lower Risk of Osteoporosis

Calcium is required to build healthy bones and is also required for the proper transmission of nerve signals between cells. If an individual does not consume enough calcium in their diet, especially if they do not ingest enough Vitamin D as well, they can develop osteoporosis, a bone disease that causes bones to become thin, brittle and break easily due to an insufficiency of calcium.

6. Fewer colds and infections

The riper the vegetables eaten, the lower the risk of colds and infections. Studies show that those who follow a vegetarian diet have only 1/3rd of the usual incidence of getting a cold as those who eat meat. The reason is that approximately 80% of colds can be prevented by proper nutrition. Many cooked vegetables are known to inhibit viruses and bacteria, such as fermented vegetables like kimchi and sauerkraut, which also act as a probiotic to help maintain healthy gut flora.

I hope this book has inspired you to make a change in your diet and lifestyle but the biggest change will be when you start having the body you want to see.

The more we do for ourselves, the more we have control over our lives, our health, and our future.

Good luck!

CPSIA information can be obtained
at www.ICGtesting.com
Printed in the USA
BVHW091514180621
609897BV00002B/94